KIDNEY TRANSPLANT COOKBOOK

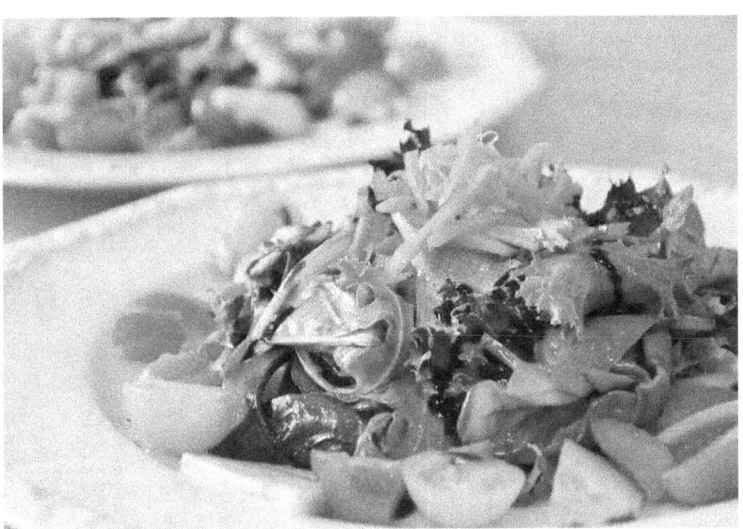

DR. MAUREEN MOORE

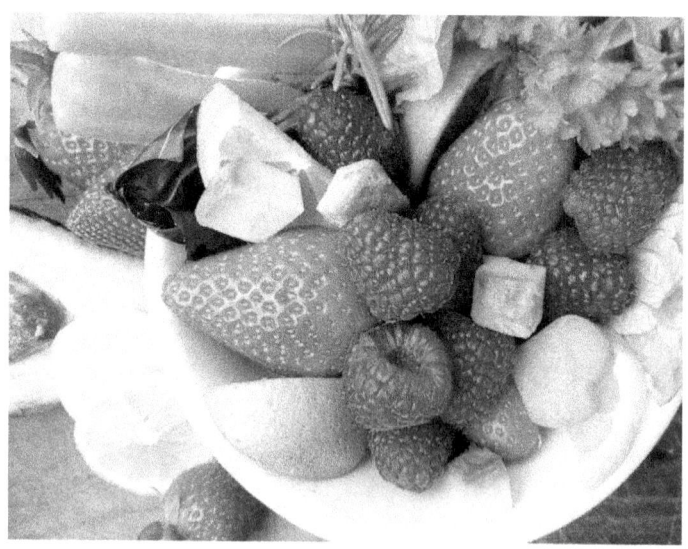

TABLE OF CONTENT

CHAPTER ONE

Introduction

Kidney transplant, a medical marvel and life-altering procedure, stands as a beacon of hope for individuals grappling with end-stage renal disease (ESRD) or other severe kidney disorders.

This intricate and transformative medical intervention involves the surgical transplantation of a healthy kidney from a living or deceased donor into the recipient, offering the promise of renewed vitality and improved quality of life.

The kidneys, vital organs responsible for filtering waste and excess fluids from the blood, play a crucial role in maintaining the body's overall balance.

When these organs fail due to conditions such as chronic kidney disease (CKD) or genetic disorders, the resulting decline in kidney function necessitates advanced medical interventions. Kidney transplant emerges as a definitive solution, holding the potential to restore normal kidney function and liberate individuals from the constraints of dialysis.

This comprehensive guide to kidney transplant delves into the multifaceted aspects of this life-changing procedure.

From the initial stages of evaluation and donor compatibility assessment to the intricacies of the surgical process and post-transplant care, each phase of the kidney transplant journey is explored in detail.

Key Components:

Patient Evaluation: Unravel the meticulous process of patient evaluation, where medical professionals assess the physical, emotional, and psychological suitability of individuals for transplantation.

This stage involves an exhaustive examination of medical history, compatibility testing, and discussions about the potential risks and benefits.

Donor Selection: Gain insights into the critical aspect of donor selection, examining the criteria for identifying suitable living or deceased donors. The guide explores the ethical considerations, evaluation procedures, and the compassionate act of altruistic kidney donation.

Surgical Procedure: Delve into the intricacies of the surgical procedure, from the careful removal of the donor kidney to the precise implantation in the recipient. Understand the advancements in surgical techniques that contribute to enhanced outcomes and reduced recovery times.

Post-Transplant Care: Navigate the crucial phase of post-transplant care, where meticulous monitoring, immunosuppressive medications, and lifestyle adjustments are pivotal to ensure the success of the transplant and long-term well-being.

Challenges and Triumphs: Explore the potential challenges and triumphs that individuals may encounter on their post-transplant journey. From the joys of restored independence to the ongoing management of potential complications, this guide provides a comprehensive overview.

Kidney transplant represents not only a medical intervention but a profound opportunity for a renewed lease on life.

This guide serves as a companion for patients, their families, and the medical community, offering valuable insights into the intricacies of kidney transplantation and the transformative impact it can have on the lives of those who embark on this remarkable journey.

Benefits of Kidney Transplant

Kidney transplant, as a definitive treatment for end-stage renal disease (ESRD) or severe kidney disorders, offers a multitude of benefits that significantly impact the quality of life and overall well-being of individuals. Here are some key benefits associated with kidney transplant:

Renewed Quality of Life: Kidney transplant often leads to a substantial improvement in the quality of life for recipients. With restored kidney function, individuals can experience increased energy levels, improved appetite, and a reduction in symptoms associated with kidney failure, such as fatigue and difficulty concentrating.

Elimination of Dialysis Dependence: For individuals undergoing regular dialysis due to kidney failure, transplant provides a chance to break free from the constraints of this life-sustaining but demanding procedure.

Transplant recipients can resume a more normal daily routine without the time-consuming and restrictive schedule of dialysis treatments.

Improved Long-Term Survival: Studies consistently show that kidney transplant recipients generally experience better long-term survival rates compared to individuals remaining on dialysis. The transplant helps mitigate the risks associated with complications of kidney failure and its impact on overall health.

Enhanced Cardiovascular Health: Kidney transplant is associated with improved cardiovascular health.

As the transplanted kidney restores proper fluid and electrolyte balance, it contributes to better blood pressure control and reduced cardiovascular risk factors, leading to a lower incidence of heart-related complications.

Nutritional Well-being: Transplant recipients often experience improvements in their nutritional status. The restored kidney function allows for better regulation of essential minerals and nutrients in the body, addressing issues like anemia and bone health that can be compromised in advanced kidney disease.

Freedom from Dietary Restrictions: Kidney transplant recipients may enjoy more dietary freedom compared to individuals on dialysis.

While they still need to maintain a healthy lifestyle, including a balanced diet and regular exercise, they often have fewer dietary restrictions, contributing to a more enjoyable and varied eating experience.

Increased Independence: Post-transplant, individuals often regain a sense of independence.

They are no longer tied to a dialysis schedule, allowing for more flexibility in work, travel, and daily activities. This increased autonomy positively influences mental well-being and overall life satisfaction.

Psychosocial Benefits: Kidney transplant can have positive psychosocial impacts, improving mental health and emotional well-being. Patients often experience reduced anxiety, depression, and a greater sense of normalcy, contributing to an overall positive outlook on life.

Potential for Family Planning: For individuals of childbearing age, kidney transplant opens the possibility of family planning without the challenges and risks associated with pregnancy in the context of kidney failure and dialysis.

Economic Impact: While there are initial costs and potential ongoing expenses related to immunosuppressive medications and follow-up care, kidney transplant can be cost-effective in the long run compared to the ongoing expenses of dialysis treatments.

It's important to note that while kidney transplant offers numerous benefits, it also comes with potential risks and requires ongoing medical management. Patient outcomes can vary, and the decision to undergo transplantation should be made in consultation with healthcare professionals, considering individual health factors and circumstances.

Causes of Kidney Trabsplant

Kidney transplantation is typically considered as a treatment option for individuals with end-stage renal disease (ESRD) or other severe kidney disorders. The primary causes that may lead someone to undergo a kidney transplant include:

Chronic Kidney Disease (CKD): Progression of chronic kidney disease, often caused by conditions such as diabetes, hypertension, glomerulonephritis, or polycystic kidney disease, can eventually lead to end-stage renal disease. When the kidneys fail to function adequately, transplantation becomes a viable treatment option.

Hypertensive Nephropathy: Prolonged and uncontrolled high blood pressure can lead to damage to the small blood vessels in the kidneys, a condition known as hypertensive nephropathy. This can contribute to chronic kidney disease and, in some cases, necessitate a kidney transplant.

Diabetic Nephropathy: Diabetes, particularly when poorly controlled over an extended period, can cause damage to the kidneys. Diabetic nephropathy is a common cause of end-stage renal disease, prompting consideration for kidney transplantation.

Polycystic Kidney Disease (PKD): Inherited conditions such as polycystic kidney disease involve the development of fluid-filled cysts in the kidneys, leading to a decline in kidney function over time. For individuals with advanced PKD, kidney transplant may be recommended.

Glomerulonephritis: Inflammation of the glomeruli, the filtering units of the kidneys, can result in glomerulonephritis. This condition, whether acute or chronic, may lead to kidney damage and the need for transplantation.

Congenital Abnormalities: Some individuals are born with structural or functional abnormalities in their kidneys. Severe congenital kidney disorders may require transplantation for optimal long-term outcomes.

Inherited Kidney Disorders: Certain genetic conditions can predispose individuals to kidney disease, often leading to progressive decline in kidney function. In some cases, kidney transplantation becomes necessary to address the underlying genetic disorder.

Recurrent Kidney Stones: Persistent and recurrent kidney stones, particularly when they cause structural damage to the kidneys, may lead to chronic kidney disease and the eventual need for transplantation.

Infections: Severe and recurrent kidney infections, if left untreated or if they lead to irreversible kidney damage, may necessitate transplantation.

Trauma or Injury: Trauma or injury to the kidneys, such as severe accidents or blunt force trauma, may result in irreversible damage, leading to the need for transplantation.

It's important to note that kidney transplantation is a complex medical procedure, and the decision to undergo transplantation is typically made in consultation with healthcare professionals.

Patient eligibility for transplantation is assessed based on factors such as overall health, compatibility with potential donors, and the severity of kidney disease.

The availability of suitable donors, whether living or deceased, also plays a crucial role in the feasibility of kidney transplantation.

Symptoms of Kidney Transplant

After undergoing a kidney transplant, recipients may experience various symptoms during the post-transplant period.

It's important to note that while some symptoms are common as the body adjusts to the new kidney, others may indicate potential complications that require medical attention. Here are both normal post-transplant symptoms and potential signs of complications:

Normal Post-Transplant Symptoms:

Fatigue: Feeling tired or having low energy levels is common as the body adjusts to the changes.

Pain: Mild discomfort or pain at the surgical site is expected initially, but this should gradually improve over time.

Swelling: Swelling around the surgical area or in the legs may occur but should diminish as healing progresses.

Bruising: Some bruising around the incision site is normal and typically resolves with time.

Changes in Urination: Initial changes in urine color and frequency are normal as the transplanted kidney begins to function.

Weight Gain: Some weight gain may occur due to fluid retention, but this is often temporary.

Changes in Medication: Adjustment of immunosuppressive medications may lead to side effects such as changes in blood pressure, glucose levels, or mood.

Potential Signs of Complications:

Fever: Persistent or high fever may indicate an infection and should be reported to healthcare providers.

Painful Urination: Pain or discomfort during urination may signal a urinary tract infection.

Decreased Urine Output: A sudden decrease in urine output may indicate issues with kidney function.

Swelling and Fluid Retention: Severe or worsening swelling, particularly in the face or extremities, may suggest fluid overload.

Signs of Rejection: Symptoms of kidney rejection can include decreased urine output, swelling, and increased blood pressure. Regular follow-up appointments and monitoring are crucial to detect rejection early.

High Blood Pressure: Persistent or significantly elevated blood pressure should be addressed promptly.

Changes in Medication Response: If side effects from immunosuppressive medications become severe or intolerable, it's essential to consult healthcare providers.

Signs of Infection: Symptoms such as persistent cough, difficulty breathing, or other signs of infection should be evaluated promptly.

CHAPTER TWO

KIDNEY TRANSPLANT RECIPES

Recipe 1: Grilled Lemon Herb Chicken

Ingredients:

3 boneless, skinless chicken breasts

1 tablespoon olive oil

1 lemon (juiced)

2 cloves garlic (minced)

1 teaspoon dried oregano

1 teaspoon dried thyme

Salt and pepper to taste

Instructions:

In a bowl, mix olive oil, lemon juice, minced garlic, dried oregano, dried thyme, salt, and pepper to create a marinade.

Place the chicken breasts in a resealable plastic bag or shallow dish and pour the marinade over them. Seal or cover and refrigerate for at least 30 minutes.

Preheat the grill to medium-high heat.

Remove the chicken from the marinade and grill for 6-8 minutes per side or until fully cooked.

Allow the chicken to rest for a few minutes before serving.

Cooking Time: Approximately 15-20 minutes

Recipe 2: Quinoa and Vegetable Salad

Ingredients:

1 cup quinoa, rinsed

2 cups water or low-sodium vegetable broth

1 cup cherry tomatoes, halved

1 cucumber, diced

1 bell pepper, diced

1/4 cup red onion, finely chopped

2 tablespoons fresh parsley, chopped

2 tablespoons olive oil

2 tablespoons balsamic vinegar

Salt and pepper to taste

Instructions:

In a medium saucepan, combine quinoa and water or broth. Bring to a boil, then reduce heat, cover, and simmer for 15-20 minutes or until quinoa is cooked and water is absorbed.

Fluff quinoa with a fork and let it cool to room temperature.

In a large bowl, combine quinoa, cherry tomatoes, cucumber, bell pepper, red onion, and parsley.

In a small bowl, whisk together olive oil, balsamic vinegar, salt, and pepper. Pour the dressing over the salad and toss to combine.

Refrigerate for at least 30 minutes before serving.

Cooking Time: Approximately 20-25 minutes (including cooling time)

Recipe 3: Baked Salmon with Dill

Ingredients:

3 salmon fillets

2 tablespoons olive oil

1 lemon (sliced)

2 tablespoons fresh dill, chopped

Salt and pepper to taste

Instructions:

Preheat the oven to 375°F (190°C).

Place the salmon fillets on a baking sheet lined with parchment paper.

Drizzle olive oil over the salmon and season with salt, pepper, and chopped dill.

Place lemon slices on top of each fillet.

Bake for 15-20 minutes or until the salmon flakes easily with a fork.

Cooking Time: Approximately 15-20 minutes

Recipe 4: Lentil and Vegetable Soup

Ingredients:

1 cup dried green or brown lentils, rinsed

4 cups low-sodium vegetable broth

1 onion, diced

2 carrots, diced

2 celery stalks, diced

2 cloves garlic, minced

1 teaspoon cumin

1 teaspoon paprika

Salt and pepper to taste

2 tablespoons olive oil

Fresh parsley for garnish (optional)

Instructions:

In a large pot, heat olive oil over medium heat. Add diced onion, carrots, celery, and minced garlic. Sauté until vegetables are softened.

Add lentils, vegetable broth, cumin, paprika, salt, and pepper. Bring to a boil, then reduce heat and simmer for 25-30 minutes or until lentils are tender.

Adjust seasoning if necessary. Serve hot, garnished with fresh parsley if desired.

Cooking Time: Approximately 35-40 minutes

Recipe 5: Roasted Vegetable Medley

Ingredients:

2 cups cauliflower florets

2 cups broccoli florets

2 carrots, sliced

1 red bell pepper, sliced

2 tablespoons olive oil

1 teaspoon dried thyme

1 teaspoon garlic powder

Salt and pepper to taste

Instructions:

Preheat the oven to 400°F (200°C).

In a large bowl, toss cauliflower, broccoli, carrots, and red bell pepper with olive oil, dried thyme, garlic powder, salt, and pepper.

Spread the vegetables in a single layer on a baking sheet.

Roast in the oven for 25-30 minutes or until the vegetables are tender and slightly browned.

Serve as a side dish or over a bed of quinoa or rice.

Cooking Time: Approximately 25-30 minutes

Recipe 6: Berry and Spinach Salad with Balsamic Vinaigrette

Ingredients:

3 cups fresh spinach leaves, washed

1 cup mixed berries (strawberries, blueberries, raspberries)

1/4 cup feta cheese, crumbled (optional)

1/4 cup walnuts, chopped

2 tablespoons balsamic vinegar

1 tablespoon olive oil

1 teaspoon honey

Salt and pepper to taste

Instructions:

In a large bowl, combine fresh spinach, mixed berries, feta cheese, and chopped walnuts.

In a small bowl, whisk together balsamic vinegar, olive oil, honey, salt, and pepper to create the vinaigrette.

Drizzle the vinaigrette over the salad and toss gently to coat.

Serve immediately as a refreshing and nutritious salad option.

Preparation Time: Approximately 15-20 minutes

Recipe 7: Turkey and Vegetable Stir-Fry

Ingredients:

1 pound lean turkey breast, thinly sliced

2 cups broccoli florets

1 red bell pepper, sliced

1 yellow bell pepper, sliced

1 cup snap peas, trimmed

2 tablespoons low-sodium soy sauce

1 tablespoon olive oil

1 teaspoon ginger, minced

2 cloves garlic, minced

1 tablespoon sesame seeds (optional)

Brown rice or cauliflower rice for serving

Instructions:

In a wok or large skillet, heat olive oil over medium-high heat.

Add turkey slices and cook until browned and cooked through.

Add broccoli, red and yellow bell peppers, snap peas, ginger, and garlic. Stir-fry for 5-7 minutes until vegetables are tender-crisp.

Drizzle soy sauce over the stir-fry and toss to combine.

Sprinkle with sesame seeds if desired. Serve over brown rice or cauliflower rice.

Cooking Time: Approximately 20-25 minutes

Recipe 8: Sweet Potato and Black Bean Salad

Ingredients:

2 medium sweet potatoes, peeled and diced

1 can (15 oz) black beans, drained and rinsed

1 red onion, finely chopped

1/4 cup fresh cilantro, chopped

2 tablespoons olive oil

1 lime (juiced)

1 teaspoon ground cumin

Salt and pepper to taste

Instructions:

Steam or boil sweet potato cubes until tender but still firm. Allow them to cool.

In a large bowl, combine sweet potatoes, black beans, red onion, and cilantro.

In a small bowl, whisk together olive oil, lime juice, ground cumin, salt, and pepper. Pour over the salad and toss gently to coat.

Refrigerate for at least 30 minutes before serving.

Preparation Time: Approximately 25-30 minutes

Recipe 9: Lemon Garlic Shrimp Skewers

Ingredients:

1 pound large shrimp, peeled and deveined

Zest of 1 lemon

Juice of 1 lemon

2 tablespoons olive oil

2 cloves garlic, minced

1 teaspoon dried oregano

Salt and pepper to taste

Wooden skewers, soaked in water

Instructions:

Preheat the grill or grill pan.

In a bowl, combine lemon zest, lemon juice, olive oil, minced garlic, dried oregano, salt, and pepper to create a marinade.

Thread shrimp onto soaked skewers and brush with the marinade.

Grill shrimp skewers for 2-3 minutes per side or until they are opaque and cooked through.

Serve hot, garnished with fresh herbs if desired.

Cooking Time: Approximately 8-10 minutes

Recipe 10: Egg and Vegetable Frittata

Ingredients:

6 large eggs

1 cup cherry tomatoes, halved

1 cup spinach, chopped

1/2 cup red bell pepper, diced

1/4 cup feta cheese, crumbled

1 tablespoon olive oil

1 teaspoon dried oregano

Salt and pepper to taste

Instructions:

Preheat the oven to 375°F (190°C).

In a bowl, whisk together eggs, dried oregano, salt, and pepper.

In an oven-safe skillet, heat olive oil over medium heat. Add cherry tomatoes, spinach, and red bell pepper, sautéing until the vegetables are softened.

Pour the whisked eggs over the vegetables in the skillet.

Sprinkle crumbled feta cheese over the top.

Transfer the skillet to the preheated oven and bake for 15-20 minutes or until the frittata is set and lightly browned.

Slice and serve warm.

Cooking Time: Approximately 25-30 minutes

Recipe 11: Chicken and Vegetable Kebabs

Ingredients:

1 pound boneless, skinless chicken breasts, cut into cubes

1 zucchini, sliced

1 yellow squash, sliced

1 red onion, sliced

Cherry tomatoes

2 tablespoons olive oil

1 teaspoon dried rosemary

1 teaspoon garlic powder

Salt and pepper to taste

Wooden skewers, soaked in water

Instructions:

Preheat the grill or grill pan.

In a bowl, mix olive oil, dried rosemary, garlic powder, salt, and pepper.

Thread chicken cubes, zucchini, yellow squash, red onion, and cherry tomatoes onto the soaked skewers.

Brush the kebabs with the olive oil and herb mixture.

Grill for 10-15 minutes, turning occasionally, until the chicken is cooked through and the vegetables are tender.

Cooking Time: Approximately 15-20 minutes

Recipe 12: Greek Yogurt Parfait with Berries

Ingredients:

1 cup Greek yogurt

1/2 cup mixed berries (blueberries, strawberries, raspberries)

2 tablespoons honey

1/4 cup granola

1 tablespoon chopped nuts (almonds, walnuts)

Fresh mint leaves for garnish (optional)

Instructions:

In a glass or bowl, layer Greek yogurt at the bottom.

Add a layer of mixed berries on top of the yogurt.

Drizzle honey over the berries.

Sprinkle granola and chopped nuts over the honey.

Repeat the layers if desired.

Garnish with fresh mint leaves.

Serve chilled.

Preparation Time: Approximately 10-15 minutes

Recipe 13: Spinach and Mushroom Stuffed Chicken Breast

Ingredients:

4 boneless, skinless chicken breasts

2 cups fresh spinach, chopped

1 cup mushrooms, finely chopped

1/2 cup low-fat mozzarella cheese, shredded

2 cloves garlic, minced

1 tablespoon olive oil

1 teaspoon dried thyme

Salt and pepper to taste

Instructions:

Preheat the oven to 375°F (190°C).

In a skillet, heat olive oil over medium heat. Add garlic, spinach, and mushrooms. Sauté until the vegetables are tender.

Butterfly each chicken breast and stuff with the sautéed spinach and mushroom mixture.

Sprinkle each chicken breast with shredded mozzarella, dried thyme, salt, and pepper.

Place the stuffed chicken breasts in a baking dish and bake for 25-30 minutes or until the chicken is cooked through.

Cooking Time: Approximately 30-35 minutes

Recipe 14: Quinoa-Stuffed Bell Peppers

Ingredients:

4 bell peppers, halved and seeds removed

1 cup quinoa, cooked

1 can (15 oz) black beans, drained and rinsed

1 cup corn kernels (fresh or frozen)

1 cup cherry tomatoes, diced

1/2 cup red onion, finely chopped

1 teaspoon ground cumin

1 teaspoon chili powder

Salt and pepper to taste

Fresh cilantro for garnish (optional)

Instructions:

Preheat the oven to 375°F (190°C).

In a large bowl, mix together cooked quinoa, black beans, corn, cherry tomatoes, red onion, ground cumin, chili powder, salt, and pepper.

Stuff each bell pepper half with the quinoa mixture.

Place the stuffed peppers in a baking dish and bake for 25-30 minutes or until the peppers are tender.

Garnish with fresh cilantro if desired.

Cooking Time: Approximately 30-35 minutes

Recipe 15: Baked Cod with Lemon and Herbs

Ingredients:

4 cod fillets

2 tablespoons olive oil

1 lemon (juiced)

2 tablespoons fresh parsley, chopped

1 teaspoon dried dill

Salt and pepper to taste

Instructions:

Preheat the oven to 400°F (200°C).

Place cod fillets in a baking dish.

In a small bowl, whisk together olive oil, lemon juice, chopped parsley, dried dill, salt, and pepper.

Pour the mixture over the cod fillets.

Bake for 15-20 minutes or until the cod is cooked through and flakes easily with a fork.

Cooking Time: Approximately 20-25 minutes

Recipe 16: Turkey and Vegetable Chili

Ingredients:

1 pound lean ground turkey

1 onion, chopped

2 bell peppers (any color), diced

2 cloves garlic, minced

1 can (15 oz) kidney beans, drained and rinsed

1 can (15 oz) diced tomatoes

1 cup low-sodium chicken broth

2 teaspoons chili powder

1 teaspoon cumin

1 teaspoon paprika

Salt and pepper to taste

Fresh cilantro for garnish (optional)

Instructions:

In a large pot, cook ground turkey over medium heat until browned.

Add chopped onion, bell peppers, and minced garlic. Sauté until vegetables are softened.

Stir in kidney beans, diced tomatoes, chicken broth, chili powder, cumin, paprika, salt, and pepper.

Bring the mixture to a boil, then reduce heat and simmer for 20-25 minutes.

Garnish with fresh cilantro before serving.

Cooking Time: Approximately 30-35 minutes

Recipe 17: Shrimp and Avocado Salad

Ingredients:

1-pound large shrimp, peeled and deveined

2 avocados, diced

1 cup cherry tomatoes, halved

1 cucumber, diced

1/4 cup red onion, finely chopped

2 tablespoons fresh cilantro, chopped

2 tablespoons olive oil

2 tablespoons lime juice

Salt and pepper to taste

Instructions:

In a large bowl, combine diced avocados, cherry tomatoes, diced cucumber, red onion, and chopped cilantro.

In a skillet, cook shrimp with olive oil over medium-high heat until they are opaque and cooked through.

Add cooked shrimp to the salad.

Drizzle lime juice over the salad, and toss gently to combine.

Season with salt and pepper. Serve chilled.

Preparation Time: Approximately 20-25 minutes

Recipe 18: Eggplant and Tomato Bake

Ingredients:

1 large eggplant, thinly sliced

2 large tomatoes, thinly sliced

1/2 cup grated Parmesan cheese

2 tablespoons olive oil

2 teaspoons dried basil

1 teaspoon dried oregano

Salt and pepper to taste

Instructions:

Preheat the oven to 375°F (190°C).

In a baking dish, arrange alternating layers of eggplant and tomato slices.

Drizzle olive oil over the layers and sprinkle with dried basil, dried oregano, salt, and pepper.

Sprinkle grated Parmesan cheese on top.

Bake for 25-30 minutes or until the vegetables are tender and the top is golden brown.

Cooking Time: Approximately 30-35 minutes

Recipe 19: Salmon and Vegetable Skewers

Ingredients:

1 pound salmon fillets, cut into cubes

1 zucchini, sliced

1 yellow squash, sliced

1 red onion, sliced

Cherry tomatoes

2 tablespoons olive oil

1 lemon (zested and juiced)

1 teaspoon dried dill

Salt and pepper to taste

Wooden skewers, soaked in water

Instructions:

Preheat the grill or grill pan.

In a bowl, mix olive oil, lemon zest, lemon juice, dried dill, salt, and pepper.

Thread salmon cubes, zucchini, yellow squash, red onion, and cherry tomatoes onto the soaked skewers.

Brush the skewers with the olive oil and herb mixture.

Grill for 10-15 minutes, turning occasionally, until the salmon is cooked through.

Cooking Time: Approximately 15-20 minutes

Recipe 20: Quinoa and Vegetable Stir-Fry

Ingredients:

1 cup quinoa, cooked

1 cup broccoli florets

1 carrot, julienned

1 red bell pepper, sliced

1 cup snap peas, trimmed

2 tablespoons low-sodium soy sauce

1 tablespoon sesame oil

1 tablespoon rice vinegar

1 teaspoon ginger, minced

2 cloves garlic, minced

Green onions for garnish (optional)

Instructions:

In a wok or large skillet, heat sesame oil over medium-high heat.

Add ginger and garlic, stir-frying for 30 seconds.

Add broccoli, carrot, red bell pepper, and snap peas. Stir-fry for 5-7 minutes until vegetables are tender-crisp.

Add cooked quinoa to the wok.

Pour soy sauce and rice vinegar over the mixture. Toss to combine.

Garnish with chopped green onions if desired. Serve hot.

Cooking Time: Approximately 20-25 minutes

CONCLUSION

Incorporating a diverse range of kidney-friendly recipes into your culinary repertoire can not only add vibrancy to your meals but also contribute to a balanced and health-conscious lifestyle.

From grilled proteins and nutrient-rich salads to comforting stews and flavorful side dishes, these recipes prioritize ingredients that align with the needs of individuals who have undergone a kidney transplant or are managing kidney-related conditions.

Remember, personalization is key in adapting these recipes to suit individual dietary requirements and preferences.

Always consult with healthcare professionals or dietitians to ensure that these recipes align with your specific health needs. By embracing a kidney-friendly approach to cooking, you can savor delicious flavors while prioritizing your overall well-being.